Margaret Phalor Barnhart's "Journey Unknown" is an honest look at how she dealt with her journey through uncharted territory for her — breast cancer. The physical treatments are well known and provide a standard of care meant to heal. However, the emotional aspects of dealing with a cancer diagnosis are powerful and terrifying.

… I highly recommend "Journey Unknown" for each individual, but they should know that many, such as this author, have triumphantly completed the same journey.

Editorial Review for Amazon Kindle
By John McClure

★★★★★
Honest and Moving

"Sometimes when we experience pain, it is merely God's way of stretching out spaces in our heart for the joy that follows. Experiencing cancer is a painful process, both physically and emotionally. *Journey Unknown* filled my heart with joy and made me know that life's journey has been paved and made ready by God. Margaret Barnhart's brilliance, through poetry, has helped to make each day's journey more joyful for me."

Zora Kramer Brown
Founder and Chairperson
Breast Cancer Resource Committee
Washington, D.C. (1987)

"[This] book is a marvelous gift. It will be a resource to pastors and anyone who seeks to comfort and help those who are battling cancer. It will be a source of strength for anyone who undergoes surgery and treatment for cancer. I have found it to be a healing gift in my own life, and I recommend it highly."

Kenneth H. Sauer, Former Bishop
Southern Ohio Synod
Evangelical Lutheran Church in America

"… an excellent source of support for many breast cancer patients. Her words and expressions related to her journey through her episode of breast cancer over the last six years are expressed with great feeling and understanding … Meaningful and touching."

Sidney F. Miller, M.D., Director
The Ohio State University, Burn Care, Columbus, Ohio

❧

"This book gives support people insight into the process that their loved one is experiencing."

Thomas A. Nims, M.D.
Surgical Oncology, Inc., Columbus, Ohio

❧

"I've read *Journey Unknown* at least 15 times, and I still find new meaning on each page."

Mary Ann Copeland, former Executive Director,
Miami County, Ohio, American Cancer Society

"I received the book, and the day I got it, I sat down and read it cover to cover, including all the reviews, intros, etc. I seldom do that … I related to all the poems and articles, even though I didn't always have exactly the same feelings. She certainly has a gift of expression …"

Jo Anne

"*Journey Unknown* is authentic, chilling, desperate, encouraging, and victorious. You are an amazing woman; you truly live a victorious life!"

LaVerne

"A poignant expression of feelings and emotions, *Journey Unknown* paints a picture of the breast cancer experience that can be visualized and felt by all."

Susan Leigh, Oncology Nurse

Journey Unknown

Focusing on the Emotional Aspects of Cancer, Mastectomy, and Chemotherapy

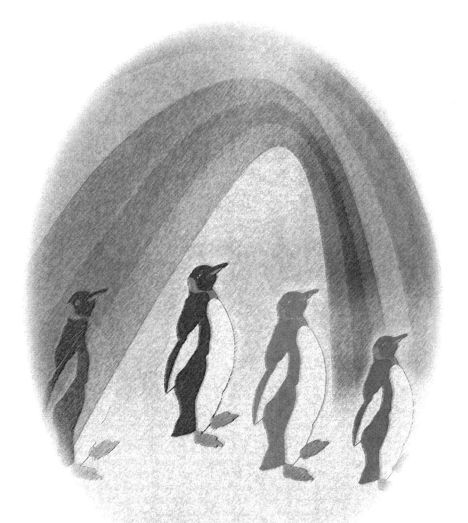

Margaret Phalor Barnhart

Journey Unknown

SECOND EDITION

by Margaret Phalor Barnhart

Illustrated by: Margaret Phalor Barnhart and Jennifer T. Cappoen
Cover Illustration: Jennifer Tipton Cappoen
Copy Editor: Nancy E. Williams

Paperback Book: ISBN: 978-0-9847683-8-7

E-Book: ISBN: 978-0-9847683-9-4

Published by Laurus Books

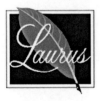

LAURUS BOOKS
P. O. Box 894
Locust Grove, GA 30248 USA
800-596-7370
www.TheLaurusCompany.com

Printed in the United States of America

This book may be purchased in both paperback and eBook from TheLaurusCompany.com, Amazon.com, BarnesandNoble.com, and other retailers around the world.

Acknowledgement

Roger Reinardy and I have never met. Twenty-five years ago, when I was on a six-month course of chemotherapy, it was his needlepoint design called "Penguin Promenade" that occupied 52 hours of my time. My eyes were weak, and I had difficulty reading. However, this needlework used larger holes with various colors of yarn. I started in the upper right corner and worked my way to the left. As the black penguins moved toward the rainbow, my mood lightened and lifted me out of depression. Roger's design was just what I needed. Recently, I was able to track him down in Minnesota and received his permission to use a rendition of his design on the cover of "Journey Unknown."

He wrote back to me, "Marge, you do me honor by taking this piece to a whole new level. Of course, you have my permission to use it on the cover of your book. My late wife was the business part of the company, and I was the design end. She would have been very happy to see our design put to such a great new use."

Thank you, dear Roger.

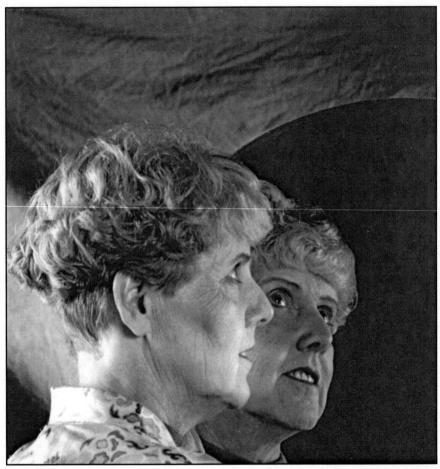

[Photo by Jim Witmer]

Note From the Author

Life's journey sent me on a search for identity and control. As a child, a daughter, and a sister, I explored and challenged. The years of education included advanced degrees in Elementary Education (Capital University), Guidance and Counseling (Miami University), and Art Therapy (Wright State University). The 28 years of my first marriage included mothering two sons, many household moves to accommodate my husband's job desires, full time work in a number of Ohio school systems, and extensive travel.

Chaos resulted when my contract as a counselor was non-renewed. I lost self-esteem and became depressed. Then I was devoured by breast cancer and its treatment. Suddenly, the accumulation of wisdom and experience was inadequate in regard to my religious beliefs and value system. 1988 was the year I was approved for disability retirement at the age of 48.

Coming back from the brink of despair, I look to the future with the light of God on my shoulder. Looking in the mirror conveys my submission to a spiritual identity and fully accepting myself as a child of God. This is the peace that passes all understanding.

Table of Contents

Foreword

In 1987, at the age of 46, Margaret Phalor Barnhart was diagnosed with breast cancer. She underwent a modified radical mastectomy, followed by six months of chemotherapy. To help ease the emotional and psychological burden of the disease and its treatment, she penned poems and sketched artwork. *Journey Unknown* is a chronological compilation of these inspirational pieces.

The book's first poem relates the awful night spent at a friend's birthday party that included three trips to the bathroom hoping the lump found in her breast earlier that day had miraculously disappeared. The penultimate poem dispels the erroneous notion that cancer is a death sentence, revealing the author's acceptance of her disease and her hope for the future. In between these two poems is an uplifting journey of one woman's battle against the physical, emotional, and psychological trauma of breast cancer. From shock, anger, and denial through depression and, finally, acceptance, Ms. Barnhart's story is powerful and touching and sure to be an inspiration to other cancer patients.

Journey Unknown can be read in its entirety in a few hours. However, the poems and artwork will certainly inspire countless hours of reflection, and the book can be re-read over and over with new insights found each time.

> OncoLink Book Review: *Journey Unknown,*
> *focusing on the emotional aspects of cancer,*
> *mastectomy, and chemotherapy*
> Kenneth Blank, MD
> University of Pennsylvania Cancer Center

Preface

Statistics can be manipulated to convey whatever message the writer chooses. They can be used to frighten, to impress, to inspire, or to prove a point. In the year 1987, I was the "one" out of the statistical eleven. There has been no recurrence.

For 46 years I was healthy and energetic, never able to appreciate the struggle of many who endure constant pain and illness. For almost two years, I was a patient in physical discomfort and emotional turmoil. I was dependent on the medical community. I was scared.

The writings and artwork contained in this book were initiated as my own therapy. When thoughts tumbled compulsively within my mind, especially at night, I sought relief through pencil and paper. I was coping with many degrees of loss, and each aspect of the illness—mastectomy, cancer, and chemotherapy—started me through the grief cycle of shock, denial, anger, bargaining, depression, and acceptance. Because these cycles were intermingled and overlapping, I often felt that I was the ball in a game of handball, never knowing which wall I would bounce from next.

"Loss" seems to be the primary issue. Loss occurs in many realms, and in order to remain psychologically healthy, every person must come to terms with their losses and find resolution.

Encouraged by my doctor to share my experiences with others, I discovered the power contained herein. Some cried. Many expressed having feelings similar to mine but from other causes. Sharing my story at such an intensely personal level was frightening. Following my first group presentation, I imaged myself as an old-fashioned camera, opened at the back, with the film exposed. I hoped I hadn't been damaged.

You, the reader, are invited to walk the path I traveled 25 years ago. If my journey becomes overwhelming, pause and reflect your thoughts and emotions through any creative means. I am convinced that the insight you gain will be well worth the effort.

Dedication

For surely I know the plans
I have for you, says the Lord,
plans for your welfare and not for harm,
to give you a future with hope.

~Jeremiah 29:11 (NRSV)

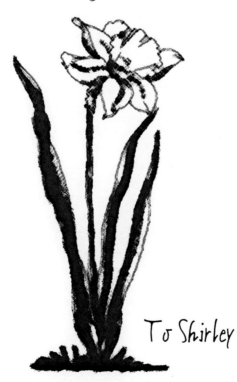

To Shirley

Elevator

A lump is an intruder in one's body. It triggers an overwhelming amount of emotion. I had been through this experience one other time, three years prior. I adamantly refused to sign consent for mastectomy, and it was not needed. (The doctor said the biopsy showed something that was a word too big and complicated for me to understand!) I was so innocent.

In January of 1987, I discovered a new lump in my breast. An antibiotic was prescribed, but after two weeks, there was no change. I was referred to a surgeon who determined that this lump was a benign cyst. More intense examination led to the discovery of another lump that was biopsied. Because of its location near the sternum, it had not shown on my last mammogram. My small town general surgeon told me if there was cancerous material found, the breast would be removed. I asked about a lumpectomy. His response was that mastectomies have been done since the 1800s and are the best treatment.

Now I had another problem. I wasn't happy with such a rigid position and told him I wanted a second opinion. He replied that he didn't know why. I was now even more convinced that I needed another perspective.

Traveling to a larger town, I received a second opinion confirming my surgeon's recommendation. The explanation was quite different. The size of the lump, the size of my breast, and the lump's proximity to my chest wall indicated clearly that I needed a modified radical mastectomy. The decision would be made while I remained under anesthesia.

The "elevator dream" occurred three days after the biopsy of tissue removed from my breast was labeled "suspicious." This dream was a powerful indicator of what was ahead. The combined sense of fear and hope was poignant. This was a recurring sensation throughout my journey.

Discovery

January

I felt the lump
　　as I showered.
In that moment
　　　the expectation
　　　　　of having fun
　　　　　　at a birthday party
　　　　　　　diminished.

Three years ago another lump
　　　was surgically removed.
　　　　Here I go again.

Should I call the doctor Monday?
Surely I'm over reacting.
Wait several weeks.
It may go away.

Socializing at the celebration
　　　was hampered by
　　　　　three trips to the bathroom
　　　　　　to feel the lump
　　　　　　　that was still there.

Elevator Dream

February

A tall city building
unfinished, under construction.
Seven stories completed.
Above them open girders.

Upon entering the elevator
I touch the button labeled "TOP."

Alone, I cling to the center pole
as surrounding buildings diminish
and city lights dim.

This upward journey
leading to the unknown
creates PANIC ...
... TERROR!

Yet, an inner peace.
A strong sense
that the elevator is connected
to a cable that I cannot see
but know is anchored.

22

Timely Concerns
March

24 hours before:
>—hospital pre-admission,
>—radical mastectomy consent form signed,
>—don't pack, but arrange items needed for personal care.

12 hours before:
>—love me, my dear, and
> hold me tight;
>—touch me and kiss me.

12 hours after:
>—Yes, I know.
>—Family surround me,
> suspend me,
>—share my burden.

24 hours after:
>—nurses hovering
>—feeling helpless
>—searching the future.

36 hours after:
>—thick gauze simulates my missing breast
>—mental rehearsal of touching the lump.

48 hours after:
>—doctor removing dressing;
>—look; see; don't think.
>—Begin to grieve this loss.

60 hours after:
>—frustrated; eating left-handed;
>—lonely; missing freedom;
>—questioning others' reactions;
>—rebelling; choosing hospital gown
>over satin and frills.

72 hours after:
>My right breast is not me,
>and yet I cry.
>But I still have the other one;
>I still have an arm and hand;
>I am still alive!

The Breakfast Tray

March

"The doctor is coming," announces the nurse,
  —coming to remove the bandages.
"Here is your breakfast," smiles an aide,
  —and swiftly goes her way.
My one-handed efforts to unseal the juice
  go unrewarded.
The clank of the cart carrying scissors
  and gauze;
The thought of cold eggs; the thought
  of swallowing;
Emotions reeling,
Eyes focus
On the breakfast tray.

Anger.

With absolute rage, I give myself permission.

Go ahead.

Push that tray away.
Send it clear across the room.

Restraint.

Smile—"Hello, Doctor!"

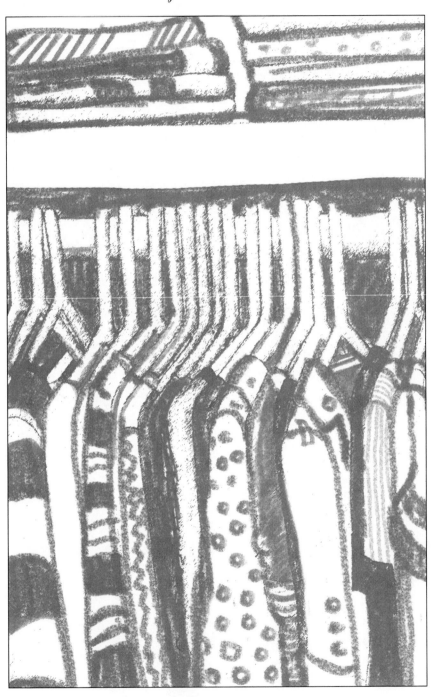

Going Home
March

Six days of hospital routine;
 —physical healing.
I've been patted and prodded,
  pampered, poked, and persuaded.
Tubes have been jerked,
 staples snipped.

I came focused on a lump.
I leave focused on a gap;
  —and statistics
  —and percentages
  —and fear of recurrence.

Going home means
  —looking in the closet
  —viewing myself through
   the eyes of others
  —leaving the cocoon.

[In 1987 insurance covered me for 6 days in hospital.]

Daffodils

Anticipating the journey home produced an unexpected fear. Although I was healing physically, I wasn't sure I could face family and friends outside the hospital setting. I had adapted well to the hospital routine.

Going home meant a return to a life I had known before the diagnosis of cancer and the amputation. I had changed radically in six days' time. The intensity of my emotions frightened me, yet I buried them inside.

Daffodils took on far greater significance than they deserved. It so happened that I was in the hospital at the time of the American Cancer Society sale of daffodils as a fund raiser. Someone had purchased them for me.

My strong feelings about carrying the daffodils the day I left the hospital intrigue me still. I had many options; yet, stoically, I held them while, at the same time, considering them a symbol that I hated. Many months later, I met the nurse who had delivered the flowers, and she recalled her uncomfortable feelings. It made us both aware of how sensitive a person may be to this diagnosis of cancer.

Six weeks later, I received daffodils in celebration of Easter. By drawing them I was able to resolve the negative thought stirred earlier. The friend who received my drawing on a note card later commented on the fact that I asked for it back. He was able to appreciate its importance to me.

I had never been on the receiving end of so much attention. The number of cards that came surprised me, and I was impressed with the careful selection of the messages. I wondered if anyone else ever experienced the negative feelings that were aroused in me.

The Yellow Daffodils

March

I didn't want the daffodils
    —a gift from an unknown donor!
I took them only to be polite.
Daffodils are supposed to be a cheerful ray,
    a yellow, delicate creation.
I wanted to deny them a place in my hands
    as I left the hospital that day.
Why hadn't I given them to the old man
    in the room next to mine?
Why was I taking them home?
Why didn't I ask my husband to carry them?

The daffodils loomed large as I sat in the
wheelchair being pushed through the corridor.
I considered dropping them in a wastebasket.
Surely, they were the label that conveyed
    the message
    that I had cancer.

My anger told me to slam them to the floor
    to be crushed under the wheels.

At home they sat in a vase.
   I hated looking at them
   and was glad when they died.

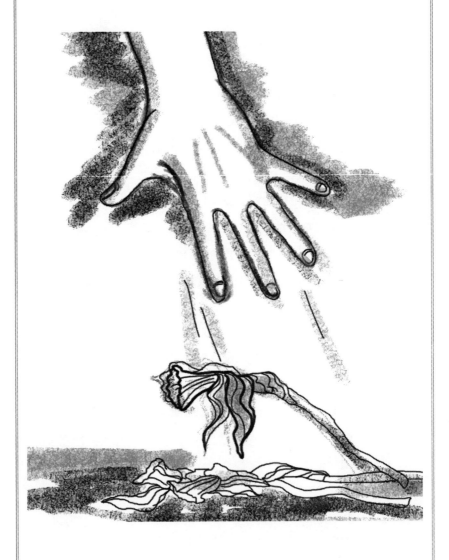

Plants, Flowers, and Cards

March

Plants, flowers, and cards
are bringing out the anger in me.
I don't want all these reminders
of my condition.
I don't want my condition.

(Mail delivery)

More cards.

Plants, flowers, and cards
help me know I am not alone.
I suffer; I'm in pain;
But enveloped by a cloud of love,
I recover.

Half a Pound of Tissue

March

Half a pound of tissue and a lump
    the size of a pea;
      —a malignant lump. Cancer.
Half a pound of tissue scooped out of its shell;
      —my breast. Nipple gone,
          skin folded over, stapled;
             muscles repositioned.

I was shown a variety of prostheses—
Almost like normal.

Sure!

Half a pound of tissue that nourished my sons
    —as many years ago
    —the nipple they sucked.
Half a pound of tissue never again
    —to be touched
    —or caressed.

Grief over half a pound of tissue?

You bet!

Drawing for a Friend
April

A daffodil drawing for you, my friend;
An Easter celebration card for you
    as you wait behind prison walls.
One for you, one for me, is my intent.
A way for me to celebrate life anew.

The daffodils of six weeks ago
    represented cancer
        and fear.
The daffodils of today,
    a resurgence,
        a rebirth.

Friend in prison,
    I think so often of the bars that
        limit you physically
            but not spiritually
        and recognize the thoughts
            and the fears
                that imprison me.

The drawing I send to you, my friend,
will be the only one made,
for my energy is spent.

Enjoy the card, my friend,
and when your need is satisfied,
would you be so kind
to return it to me?

A friend understands the request.

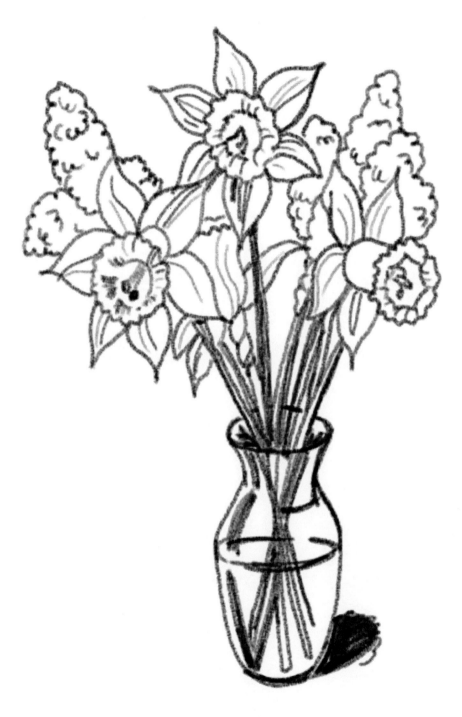

Turbulence

My decision to accept the doctor's recommendation for six months of chemotherapy sent me into a world of fear. It was unlike any I had ever experienced.

My father died of Lymphoma, and the last time I saw him, bags of chemicals were dripping into his veins. I was surprised when my mother told me that my dad had been diagnosed with Hodgkin's Disease when he was in his 40s. He had been treated with radiation and lived 35 more years before the Lymphoma diagnosis. That was encouraging.

Even so, it was very difficult for me to accept the introduction of drugs into my body.

Along with the powerful drugs was a medication intended to prevent nausea, and for me, it worked effectively throughout the six-month period. That surprised many people.

However, other side effects took their toll. The journey of the unknown led me on a turbulent path. Although I was able to work part time and maintain some other activities, there were many "down" days where I did little other than sit and sometimes work on stitchery.

A feeling that I had lost control pervaded my thoughts, and I examined the meaning of that word "control" repeatedly. My emotional state was in turmoil, with many lows and few, if any, highs. My doctor suggested I view chemotherapy as a preventive measure, like the insect spray used in a bed of flowers. That imagery helped. The loving support of many people carried me through this period.

The Chemotherapy Crisis

April

"Good news," said the surgeon.
"Lymph nodes are clear, we got
   it all."

"Not so good," says the internist,
   as two weeks after surgery
      he explains that for my type cancer
      I need at least six months
         of chemical intervention.

But I hate to experience nausea,
   and I don't want to lose my hair.

My father endured the treatment
   for a year
      before he died.

I fear the chemicals.

Do I also fear the possibility of death?

Fears and Tears
April

Listen to me, doctor,
understand my tears.

The pain of losing a breast
    has dimmed.

Fear of chemotherapy
    and unknown side effects
      immobilizes me.

Pills to take and the first IV,
    halfway through the night
      I sit,

    —afraid to fall asleep.

I want to stay awake, so
    I know I am alive.

A Hand Full of Hair
April

Three weeks of chemotherapy.
What a drag.
I need to get out—do something fun.

"Let's go to the ice show tonight,"
        suggests my husband.
Ideal.
A deal.

A shower and a quick shampoo,
A hand full of hair!
A wad of hair!

Stunning disbelief
        and simultaneous knowledge
                that I am not to be spared
                        this side effect.

Ice show, yes. Fun, no.
For, in the darkness, the audience
        cannot see the flow of tears
                cascading.

Loss of Hair
April

Is it vanity that makes me cry
　　　as my hair comes out by the handful
　　　　　three weeks after the first IV?

Or is it one more bout
　　　with the reality of cancer?

Somehow, baldness does not fit into
　　　my realm of femininity.

Shopping for a wig is drudgery.

Yes, I know.
The person is more than the body.

I know.
This, too, shall pass.

But for now,
　　　the pain is very real.

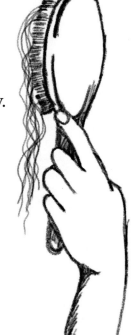

Drawing Myself
May

On this day,
        looking into a mirror,
I drew myself.

The tactile stimulation
        in the use of charcoal
                aided the process of acceptance.

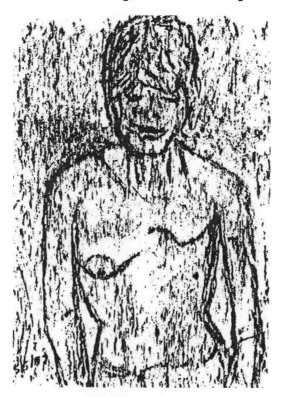

Shopping for a Breast

May

What is the proper attitude
  one assumes
      when shopping for a breast?

Naming it a prosthesis
  may be more dignified,
      but in my mind the two
          do not equate.

Just walk right up and say,
  "I need a … a … a …"

Does one confront this task
  —seriously?
  —jokingly?
  —alone?

Remember when I
  —hid behind towels?
  —coughed in church to
      avoid saying that word?
  —ordered chicken legs
      when I really wanted
      a … a … a …?

Three Reflections

May

I look in the mirror. Who am I?
In the reflection, I see
   a curly-headed blond.

Out into the world I go,
   feeling the wig
      around my head,
         wondering who notices,
            feigning confidence,
               trying to forget.

I look in the mirror. Who am I now?
   In the reflection I see
      a thin-haired old woman (my mother).

Into my world of pain I hide,
   aware of the hair loss,
      telling others it's like
         a baby's fine hair,
            trying to deny the real thoughts,
            the old woman thoughts.

I look in the mirror. Who am I now?
In the reflection, I see
   a cover-up.

Feeling my head getting cold
   in the comfort of my home,
      I add a scarf
         that offers warmth,
           that hides reality.

A scarf. And yet,
   another symbol.

Control

May

I've lost control.
I flounder.
Yet,
I sense an inward flow
    from a spiritual source
    that goes through me
    and radiates out to others
    deepening in meaning as it travels,
    continuing in its movement
    back to me
    and giving meaning to my life.

But—what do I control?

Unexpected happenings cause change
    … physical
    … emotional
    … mental
    … spiritual
    … social.

What controls me?

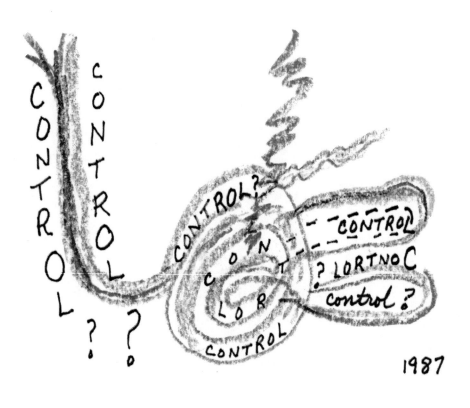

1987

Upon completion of the "control" drawing, I knew what would come next. I needed yellow!

Spiritual Insights

May

Yellow is all around me
and within me.

Yellow is spiritual.

Yellow brings peace.

Living for Today

May

I've quit fighting
—because I've given up?
—given in?
No.
It's more like giving over,
giving way.

Too much is outside my control.

I'll accept what is.
I'll live for today.

I cannot add one day to my life.
I'll do what I can for the moment.

I'll walk through the rainbow

and add color

wherever I can.

Halfway Through
July

Three months of chemo completed.
Halfway through, a relief,
    a sense of satisfaction.

Side effects a nuisance
    —exhausted, but hyper
    —numb to touch, but
        overstimulated by
        noise and light
    —metallic taste that
        explodes with spices
    —weakened vision
    —poor concentration
    —a thermostat wildly
        fluctuating;
but little nausea and
hair loss abating
I've come this far.

Facing the next IV
    —depression.
        A sense that it may never end.

Pit of my
choosing

Solid
support

Life is where
I am right now
not just at
the top

Bridges

Down
but not
out

Bottomless

People go?
Who knows this may go
where 7/15/87

Entrapment

- Negative thoughts
- Other's problems
- Lack of faith
- Looking down

55

Is it Cancer?

July

A cough, a sneeze.
    Is it normal? Or is it
        a side effect of chemotherapy?
    Or is it
        CANCER?

A headache
    different from others.
    Is it sinus? Or is it
        a side effect of chemotherapy?
    Or is it
        CANCER?

A skin mole
    not of importance before the diagnosis
        of breast cancer.
    Now it looks suspicious; yet,
        too petty to mention.
    Still a worry.
    Is it CANCER?

Will I think this way the rest of my life?
Or, after
chemotherapy ends,
will I relax?

The unanswered question still remains—
Did I have cancer?
Or …
Do I have CANCER?

Chemotherapy Miseries
August

The TASTE
… salt and spices explode within
… eat this, eat that
    seeking resolution.

The SOUND
… noises amplified
    —loading the dishwasher
    —breaking ice cubes out of trays
    —stirring sugar in the tea
    —slamming a cupboard door
… a multitude of sounds.

The TOUCH
… numbness resulting in
    —objects dropped
    —burning myself

The VISION
… looking out through inner fog
… lights at night florescent
… reading—a chore demanding
    too much energy to concentrate.

The occasional HALLUCINATION of
… gigantic
   … I mean elephantine!
      —fat tongue licking fat lips
      —eyelids stretching over enlarged eyeballs
      —huge fingers reaching out from puffy
         hands.

The SPEECH
… slowed, slurred
… searching for words
… struggling to organize thoughts.

The MUSCLES
… that tighten and cramp.

The BODY TEMPERATURE
… cold
      —shivering cold,
         … then hot
            —HOT!
               Volcanic style.

And the TIREDNESS
… I can't lie down hard enough!

THERE ARE NO GUARANTEES

- SCARED -

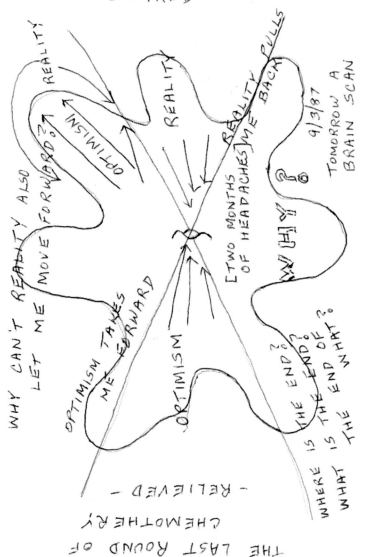

The Sixth Month
August

The end is in sight.
Five months behind me, one ahead.
Yet, each time I say "the end," I fear.

I fear the possibility—
the possibility of cancer cells
that I never knew were there,
multiplying in my body,
unaffected by drugs.

I fear the possibility—
the possibility of a need
for more chemotherapy.

I fear death by cancer—
the possibility, a possibility
I didn't accept earlier.

How can I feel excited or relieved
about a last round
when there are no guarantees
that this will always be
the last round?

Waiting for a Diagnosis
September

Yesterday, I thought I was dying
—dying of brain cancer
    as I awaited the results of a CT scan
    because of headaches
    —headaches that for two months now
        come and go.

I know someone who just died of brain cancer.

Awaiting a diagnosis can seem an eternity.
Do I plan for next week, next month?
    Is the future cancelled
    —or at least postponed?

Do I fear death, or do I fear losing life
    —or the quality of life
        to which I am accustomed?

Today, the phone call came.
CT Scan normal,
    —cause of headaches, unknown.

Headaches now seem unimportant.
Cancer cells are not the cause.

Will this fear of cancer remain forever—
   a curse
      I relentlessly bear?

Rainbow

Acceptance and resolution have involved a spiritual element I've had difficulty defining. For years I've been examining my faith and redefining my relationship with God. The artwork I relied on when at a loss for words tended to clarify the sense of connectedness. The theme occurred repeatedly beginning with the cable in the "Elevator Dream" and continuing in the "Control" drawings, appearing as the burst of light in the "Pit of my Choosing," and radiating with the penguins in their walk through the rainbow.

The journey of life is indeed unknown. In a counseling session, I was reminded that I don't need to understand life. I simply choose how to live it. Obviously, I did not choose cancer. Many of the days when I was under the influence of chemotherapy drugs, I questioned if I was capable of controlling my thoughts and emotions.

However, I was able to make many decisions along the way. I gradually became aware that as time passed and I "moved on," the focus on cancer diminished and new aspects of my life unfolded.

Push or Take it Easy?
September

The six months of chemo have ended;
I have returned to work.
Yet, life has not returned to normal.

I have such limited energy.

Do I push to keep going?

Do I take it easy as some advise?

How long do co-workers and supervisors
accept my limitations?

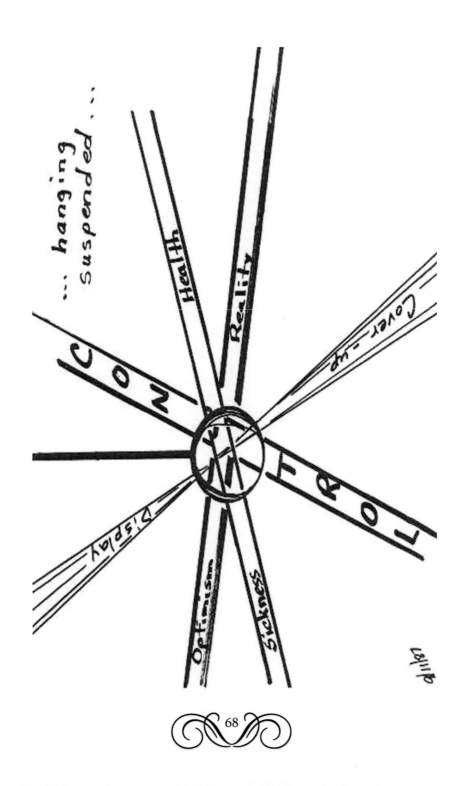

... hanging suspended ...

CONTROL

Health

Reality

Cover-up

Optimism

Sickness

Display

philip

Becoming
September

In the past I've been heard to say,
"Stitchery and needlework are not my line,
   wait until I'm old and have more time."

With chemo, I have the time.
Time to sit
   with a body that can't keep going
      and a mind that won't stop going
         and a need for a sense of control.

In and out the holes,
   needle and yarn, follow the pattern.
This I can control.

Penguins walking through a rainbow
   black and white, becoming color.
Changing.

I, too, am changing.
I can never be the same.

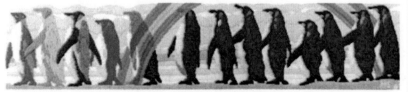

"Penguin Promenade" designed by Roger W. Reinardy • ©Horizons Designs, Inc.

Acceptance of
Loss of a Breast
September

When awakening from surgery six months ago,
   the pressing thought
      and immediate question
         centered
            on the loss of my breast.
"Is it gone?"

Acceptance has come in stages,
   overshadowed
      and submerged
         by chemotherapy.

Acceptance has come in stages
     —when the doctor removed bandages
     —when I looked … touched
     —when another looks … touches
     —when hugged.

Acceptance includes
   looking in the mirror,
      sensing the numbness,

wearing a prosthesis,
standing tall,
and most of all,
accepting
me.

Accepting Life
September

Two weeks before surgery
    and the discovery of cancer,
I told a friend I figured I had lived half my life
    at the age of 46.

Yet, in the past six months,
I've mentally and emotionally died three times
    —when I had nosebleeds,
    —when I coughed with bronchitis,
    —when the headaches were severe,
convinced that cancer was consuming me.

In this last week of chemotherapy,
my focus has been on the word "last"
    —wanting guarantees.

Acceptance relies on reality.

Six months ago,
I told my son
I didn't intend to die of cancer.

Six months ago,
with a laugh,
my son predicted
I would get hit by a car on
the way to the doctor
for my last IV.

My son was wrong.

The Paradox
September

Cancer is a life-threatening disease.
People die of cancer—
    many women,
      many men.

Having cancer
    does not mean
        I
           will die
              of cancer.

How Am I?
October

This morning I realized that
    at a meeting I attended last night,
        not one person said, "How are you?"

For eight months, I have struggled
    with an answer to that question
        because,
        for eight months, I haven't known
        how I am.

I called my doctor
    and asked, "How am I?"

"You're not sick any more!"

His response freed me—
    freed me
        to be well.

Epilogue

1988

Following my surgery and chemotherapy, I realized that all the focus had been on me. I was curious what others thought about my bout with cancer, and I sent a letter to family and close friends. You also may be interested in how things look from the other side.

February 23, 1988

Dear _____

It has been almost a year since I went into the hospital, had the mastectomy, and heard the diagnosis of breast cancer. Three weeks later, I began chemotherapy treatments that lasted for six months.

What was your reaction when you first heard the news? What thoughts led to what actions or inactions? How did you view me as I dealt with the various aspects over a long period of time? How has my experience related to your life?

Your response may be any length, any style, writing, or art work. When I publish, I'll use only your relationship to me. Your love and support have been of tremendous importance to me as I've struggled with the events of the past year.

From my husband of 26 years:

"My reaction upon first hearing the news was stunned and concerned about how you would react upon awakening from surgery. Then I wondered what effect this would have on our lives. I didn't give any thought to death, which surprises me. I was wondering how I could be supportive and do what was needed to facilitate recovery.

I tried to be more helpful, maybe a little beyond what I normally would do. I wanted to be more caring and concerned about you rather than myself. During chemo I again felt helpless and did what I could see to do. Adjustments were made, but I don't think any were dramatic."

From my oldest son: (living in another city)
"Mom, I'm too busy to write."

From my youngest son: (a senior in high school)
"Mom, I really don't have anything to say. I never thought you wouldn't make it."

From my mother:
"In mid-February, I fell and broke my leg. I had to use a walker and could not leave the house. You came to visit me and told me that you were going into the hospital to have breast surgery. You let me feel the tumor and told me what might happen. I was worried.

Your father had lymph cancer in 1948 and was given six months to live. With many prayers and x-ray therapy, he was in remission 29 years. I had been warned by the doctor that it could occur again, and this time the cancer started in the groin. Again, lymph cancer.

After 18 months of chemotherapy, he died. He was able to withstand the chemo fairly well —only a few bad reactions and several blood transfusions.

Naturally, when you told me about your impending surgery, I was really frightened. I could not be with you that day because of my broken leg.

Your sister called my neighbor and friend and asked them to come to my home to stay with me. When your husband called to tell me of your mastectomy, I broke down and was not able to talk to him. That night, after you had come out of the anesthetic, you called me, and talking to you helped calm my anxiety.

I visited you as soon as I could and was with you when your doctor called to tell you about needing six months of chemotherapy. I thought you were brave about it even though you cried as we sat there holding hands.

You withstood the chemo well, even though you were very weak and tired and had to buy a wig because you were losing your hair. Your father lost his hair three times. You seemed to get very depressed and wondered what was going to happen to you. As time went on, you improved and looked much better. You were acting more normal. I believe being able to go back to your school work and church activities, the love of your many friends and relatives, especially your husband, sons, sister and me, made it all seem easier to take.

As a mother, when one of your children hurts, you suffer with them."

From my one and only sister, six years my elder:
"Free association of my reaction—

1. fear and grief: Your husband called me at work. He was crying. I was crying. I worried about Mom and wanted to set up support for her.

2. at hospital: I felt empathy about losing a breast. I identified with that for weeks and wondered how it would be. I admired your spirit, strength, and sense of humor.

3. worried you might die: I would lose you as a friend and support person. I thought about how important you are to Mom. You would not be here to face old age with me and to help with Mom and our other relatives. I would be all alone.

4. anger about your prior depression, which I felt led to depressed immune system and, thus, cancer.

5. worried you might hate me because I'm older and should have major illness first. It's not fair.

6. worried about my daughters and wondered if this will pass to them.

7. glad that people in your community were supportive and validated your contribution to them."

From my aunt, my father's sister:

"I'm afraid I am a very poor subject to respond to your questions. I've never been one to be able to put my deepest emotions into words. I've always had a deep-seated aversion to talking about something that possibly could happen or something I truly wanted to happen. It is as though talking about it and dwelling on it will cause the reverse to happen. I always thought that I was the only one in my family that felt that way until you happened to mention that you didn't know how your Dad managed all those years without dwelling on his problem. [He and my mother never talked to each other about his cancer.] It made me realize that he must have had the same aversion.

When I first heard about your problem, I was sad that one of my favorite people had to face this trauma; then, I started thinking of all the people I knew who had gone through the same thing. Among them were two close friends who had the operation about thirty years ago and haven't slowed down since. Knowing the advances that have been made in the medical field over the past years, I was confident that, although you would have a long period of pain and discomfort to face, you would be able to handle it with your usual determination and your chin out.

The one time I really panicked was the day of your operation. Your mother told me she would call to give us the outcome as soon as she heard. When it got to be eleven o'clock that night and I hadn't heard, I was very concerned and called your sister.

As to how we view you after this shattering

experience, to us you are the same loved niece you always were. We always were very proud of your achievements and this is no exception."

From my college roommate and longtime friend:
"CANCER: the big 'C'.

HOPE – When the initial surgery was scheduled, hope filled my mind and there was no doubt but that the surgery would be minor and the tumor benign. Throughout our years of friendship, our 'group' had seemingly been immune to any major illnesses or problems. This fairy-tale existence was about to continue.

DENIAL: Calling to supposedly hear the good news brought a message of despair. This couldn't be happening—I must have heard wrong—the doctor made a mistake. If I don't think about it, it will have just been a bad dream.

QUESTIONING: Why my friend? Why not me? What is she feeling now? What thoughts does she have?

EMPATHY: Questioning and concern gave way to such strong feelings of empathy that I became, in my mind, my friend. I had pain. I tried to foresee my future and how I would deal with the diagnosis.

FRUSTRATION: Wanting so badly to be of help, to make everything whole and well again. I wanted to be in close proximity, needing to be in her company more.

HOPE: Visiting at the hospital made me aware of my friend's strength in coping, of her ability to be in control of her life, now, as she always has been. She was dealing with the situation much better than I.

QUESTIONING: Another period of questioning began and lasted for the six months of chemotherapy. Was this truly necessary? The weakness and loss of energy were almost too much to watch in a person who has always had so much drive.

We continue together in the seemingly circle of hope, unanswered questions, frustrations. We have become closer, enjoying time spent together reminiscing. Each day becomes more precious. We realize that we aren't infinite beings.

My friend's illness has made me more daring,

willing to take more risks. I want to do things now and not put them off. Together we plan a 'dream vacation' to celebrate life and God's love and grace to all of us." [Note: My three college roommates and our spouses traveled to Hawaii for a ten-day vacation.]

From my niece: (written in the third person)

" 'Oh, no!' said the girl. It had been a normal day, just like any other, until now. She had just heard that her aunt has breast cancer and is undergoing surgery that will remove one of her breasts. Her breasts! She is still so young. Is there a possibility that the cancer has spread to other parts of her body? Death! The thoughts flew wildly through the girl's head.

She had been concerned about her aunt for several years now. She was not just any relative. This aunt was special, her mother's only sister. She had known her aunt all her life. As a little girl she had gone to her aunt's wedding, and she could still remember their youthful faces. They had watched the changes through each other's lives. She had babysat her aunt's children. She had gone on vacation with their family to Washington, D.C. This aunt had shared the loss of the girl's father.

Cancer—that dirty word. Could this have been the stimulus for her aunt's recent period of depression, those hollow cheeks and the increasing loss of weight? Cancer! She must be afraid. She has worked so hard all her life, and now this. The girl felt so awful and afraid for her. She hoped the operation and the following chemotherapy treatments would be successful and not too much for her already weakened spirit and body.

The operation—her breasts! Breasts seem to mean so much to the identity of a woman. It's irrational. At the thought of losing them, the girl suddenly feels glad for what she has, even though they are small. How stupid. Our bodies. Why must we be so obsessed with our bodies?

Death—no, she is too young. This would be so awful, so unfair. The girl refused to acknowledge this possibility, but the worry persisted.

Time passes. The girl lives so far away from the ongoing trauma, yet, thinks of her aunt between

her busy hours. She sends some flowers and a card. She waits for news from her mother.

The chemotherapy begins. The strength of her aunt impresses the girl. Through all of this, her aunt continues her work and attend classes for her Master's degree. It must be better not to have time to think. She worries about her uncle's ability to adjust. Our bodies. Why always our bodies? She is losing her hair. The chemotherapy weakens her; yet, she paints a room in her house.

Time passes. She is getting better. The girl sees her aunt over the holidays. The hollowness is leaving her face. She seems to be gaining weight. The girl feels relief.

The cycle closes for the girl, but she knows that it will remain with her aunt. She is glad to hear that her aunt has begun an exercise program. It will be good for her body. Our bodies are important. It will ease her mind."

From my youngest niece:

"I believe that I am a person not easily shocked by bad news. My personal experience with disaster (accident and death of my father) and my work as a physical therapist with people who have experienced disasters (quadriplegia, stroke, M.S., etc.) have given me a more realistic or harder view of illness and death. After hearing about your previous breast cysts and knowing about your recent episode of depression, I was not shocked with the news that you had cancer and would need a radical mastectomy. I was very much saddened that you would have to deal with yet another personal hardship!

I believe I called you soon after I heard the news and offered some support. I was scared to call because I didn't know what to say. Even though I deal with people who have suffered with many different diseases and problems in the hospital setting, this situation was one I had to deal with directly on a more personal level. I would not call myself a 'huggy' person and always have to convince myself to give a hug or offer verbal support in a difficult situation. This is an area that I constantly work on since I know how much better I feel when others hug me and offer me comforting thoughts. I wish I had been able to do more for you!

Knowing that you had to have a modified radical mastectomy, I wondered how it would affect your image of yourself. I know several other women who have lost one or both breasts and appear to be functioning normally, physically and psychologically. I have not been close enough to any of these women to really help them deal with these changes in their bodies.

Looking at the psychological aspect of dealing with a medical problem such as cancer, I was concerned that you were burying yourself in so much work and activity that you didn't have time to actually face the issue. Kubler-Ross might call this time period denial, since it seemed you acted like nothing was wrong and didn't realize that your mind and body needed rest. I am glad that you have finally cut back on work and are involved in regular physical exercise. I believe that regular exercise is not only physically stimulating but psychologically uplifting as well.

The fear of cancer seems to follow us wherever

we go. We constantly hear speculation on causes and very little on cure. Over Christmas I had my first taste of that fear for myself. When I developed abnormally swollen glands throughout my body, I immediately thought of Hodgkin's Disease. Well, I let the doctor know my fears and was thankful to find out it was only an allergy to sulfa medication. This experience made me realize how vulnerable we all are to the fear of the unknown."

From the friend who had a birthday party:

"My first reaction was fear for the life of my dear friend. I had just been through a scare with the same physical problem and hoped yours would end in the same negative report I had gotten.

I internalized feelings and wondered if I would be next. A natural reaction, I suppose.

My next reaction was what I could do to help you get through this difficulty and reach the other side to be healthy again. I found what was important was to listen to you at the various stages – trying to be an active listener."

From the friend who was in prison:

"As I reflect back on a year ago, I recall your first letter informing me of your surgery and pending recuperation. My first remembrance was that I said to myself, 'Oh my God, what else does she have to face? Enough is enough. Why her?'

I then felt a closer kinship with you as I related it to my situation; indeed, I've faced a different cancer – less externally obvious but nonetheless real. It, too, had to be treated before wellness was possible. If not treated, it might have also spread. At that time, I had been in therapy for close to a year and had passed through much self-searching. I related to your experiences through mine, translated into physical and spiritual terms and felt empathy. I hope that has shown through in my letters to you.

I think the thing that touched me most deeply might be considered a small thing. You shared the card (drawing) you did of the daffodils and then asked me to return it to you after a while. It was like having a great masterpiece on display at my home, on loan. It meant much to me because I knew how much effort it took to accomplish this visual expression.

I felt over the long haul we both grew to a deeper understanding of each other as fellow human beings along life's road. You have shared inner feelings with me as I have with you. For me it only can enhance my appreciation of your victories because I have been privileged to walk with you through the battles and near defeats. Your struggles have helped me in part face my own inadequacies and added some strength to my endeavors. I feel quite comfortable being called a friend along life's way."

MY RESPONSE – 1988

"There is no adequate way to say thank you to you, my family and friends. As I look at each response, I am aware of the effort required to answer my questions. I am impressed with the thoughtfulness given to this task. When I received and read each letter, there was an overwhelming sense of love and strength that radiated into the depths of my being. Thank you."

When I read through the responses as a collection, I was fascinated with the overlapping and interweaving of themes. They coincided to a great degree with many of the feelings that I expressed in *Journey Unknown*. The support that is so evident carried me into the next phase of my unknown journey with even greater strength.

While recuperating from the mastectomy, my oldest son was diagnosed with mononucleosis and wanted to come home. He took one sofa, and I took the other. We didn't talk about cancer, and that was okay.

My youngest son was a high school senior, busy with school activities. One evening after I was told I would need chemotherapy, I was in a daze. There was a half-finished puzzle on the dining room table, and I sat down to work on it. He joined me. That was when I told him I didn't intend to die of cancer. His response was that "I'd probably get hit by a car on the way to my doctor's office for my last IV."

Depression continued to be a major problem, and even though I was taking medication, the inability to work, coupled with the gray days of Ohio, took their toll. I sought counseling from my pastor, and he led me down a destructive path, adding more stress to my life. My first marriage wasn't strong enough to endure and ended in divorce. Ultimately, years of professional therapy helped me get back on my feet.

One day as I waited in my car for a traffic light to turn from red to green, I watched a squirrel on a telephone wire that went across the street high above my head. The tiny gray squirrel scampered a third of the way across and began to fall. I watched curiously as it righted itself and continued on. Suddenly it toppled again, yet held on to the wire and righted itself once more. I hoped traffic would not force me to move on before this drama was complete. Would you believe this squirrel lost its balance again? This time I laughed and was amazed to see it complete the journey upside down on that flimsy wire. I realized that, in that position, one can only look up.

My life since 1987 has been much like that of the squirrel. While I survived the cancer, the treatment caused ongoing problems. Over the years doctors have thought I had a mild, non-paralytic form of polio as a child, and that would explain why chemotherapy substantially weakened my legs.

Working as an elementary school counselor required me to be up and down the staircase numerous times a day. Sometimes I stood at the bottom, looking up, not sure I had the strength to go to the third floor where my office was located.

When I couldn't hear the children's voices, evaluation showed hearing loss in the middle ear —the tiny bones had calcified. There were days when I would make a phone call and repeat it a half hour later, with no recall. The problems of the children and their families overwhelmed me. Ultimately, I was placed on disability retirement.

TWENTY-FIVE YEARS LATER – 2012

A generation later!

My mother, aunt, and first husband have passed on. My sister and nieces are a very important part of my life. My oldest son is married and has an adult son. My youngest son is married and has a ten-year-old daughter. My college friend is busy with her family. We see each other when possible.

I don't think about cancer much anymore. A mammogram can raise my heartbeat but has always been a blip on my radar. I married Charlie in 1992. He had been my masseur for three years. Following divorce from my first husband, we began to date. He taught me to say, "I love you." That had been lacking in my life to that point. Now, my sons and their families speak of love with their wives and children. My heart swells. Charlie never fails to express his love to his daughter, three grandchildren, and the great-grandchildren. And now, I have learned to do the same.

We have been married twenty years and have lived in Arizona since 1998. Blue skies and a

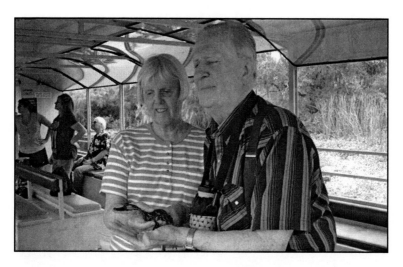

warmer climate are very important to my well-being. The dry air of the desert lessens the pain of arthritis. The hard part is that all of our family members are in the East.

Charlie is totally blind and has been since he was ten years old. A virus destroyed his optic nerve. Even so, he is quite independent. Living in Tucson has worked well for us. He has door to door transportation and activities for the visually impaired. He makes the bed, does the laundry (after I sort it), manages the dishwasher, takes the garbage out, and any other household chore I can think of.

I find it quite amusing that we married. When

I was a freshman in college, I dated a guy who had been blind since birth. After our third date my mother said, "You aren't going to marry a blind man are you?" What did I do? I married a blind man. Mom adjusted, and one time when she was visiting, she asked Charlie for a massage! My mother?

When I was a substitute teacher, I encountered a fourth grade girl who had been blind since birth. She had her Braille textbooks, Braille writer and typewriter at her desk. I had no training or experience teaching a student who was blind. We were scheduled to play volleyball for phys ed. Concerned for her safety, I asked her to help me keep score. She walked out of the gym and went home to her mother. She wanted to play volleyball, and her mother said it was OK. She taught me not to assume and to ask her how she will know where the ball is.

Many years later, a teacher who is blind, taught me even more. She taught a class for the blind and visually impaired and helped me understand that blindness limits a person in some ways but not all ways. There are other ways of seeing. She had a guide dog and owned her own home. We became friends and ate out together frequently. She asked me to please let her know when she encountered something on her plate that she couldn't see, such as the anchovy in a Greek salad or a blob of butter on the pancakes.

My lack of stamina and a back injury prevent me from accomplishing the many challenges my brain dreams up. Body weakness keeps bringing me back to a reality I still have difficulty accepting. Leading adult Christian small groups has allowed me to use my education and experience. I also facilitate groups and speak to audiences with an interest in breast cancer.

THE DAFFODIL STORY

The day I was discharged from the hospital, I took with me a bouquet of daffodils. To me, they were a symbol that I had cancer because they had been purchased from a fund-raiser of our local American Cancer Society. I carried them stoically even though I did not want them.

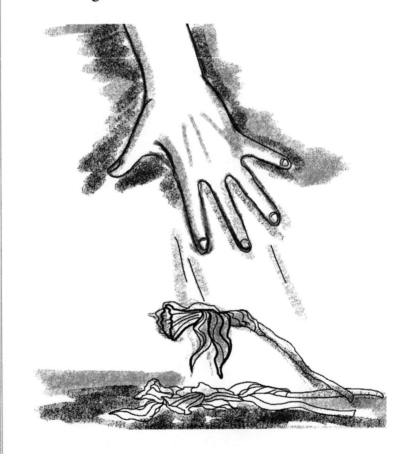

Easter arrived and someone gave me a bouquet of daffodils and hyacinths. They were beautiful sitting on my kitchen table, especially when the sun shone on them. Two weeks later, they died.

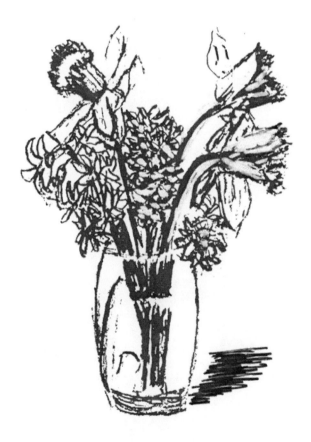

The day I saw daffodils growing in a neighbor's garden, I immediately knew these were the flowers with the most meaning. These daffodils were rooted in the earth. Although they would die, they would rise again in a year.

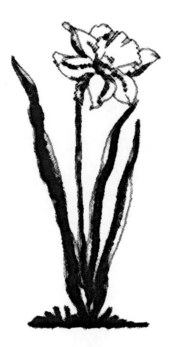

Because of this garden daffodil, I decided to dedicate *Journey Unknown* to Shirley, my therapist. She played a large role in my healing and recovery.

I rest in the arms of God, the Creator, who brought order out of chaos. God reigns—robed in majesty, girded with strength. He is mightier than the waves of the sea, yet, gentle enough to cradle a baby.

I believe God placed his Son on this earth so I could learn from Him. God sacrificed His Son for me, just as the prophets foretold.

I believe God intervenes in my mind, gives me ideas, and helps me make decisions. He leads others into my path and leads me into the paths of others. He shows me his love and the way of peace.

I view my life as a stage, a span. And I view death as a transition to another existence that God, in infinite wisdom, has also designed.

I Was There to Hear Your Borning Cry

~John Ylvisaker

I was there to hear your borning cry,
I'll be there when you are old.
I rejoiced the day you were baptized,
to see your life unfold.

I was there when you were but a child,
with a faith to suit you well;
in a blaze of light you wandered off
to find where demons dwell.

When you heard the wonder of the word
I was there to cheer you on;
you were raised to praise the living Lord,
to whom you now belong.

If you find someone to share your time
and you join your hearts as one,
I'll be there to make your verses rhyme
from dusk till rising sun.

In the middle ages of your life,
not too old, no longer young,
I'll be there to guide you through the night,
complete what I've begun.

When the evening gently closes in
and you shut your weary eyes,
I'll be there as I have always been
with just one more surprise.

I was there to hear your borning cry,
I'll be there when you are old.
I rejoiced the day you were baptized,
to see your life unfold.

CPSIA information can be obtained at www.ICGtesting.com
Printed in the USA
BVOW072040050412

287004BV00003B/9/P